Winning Weight Loss
For Teens

Winning Weight Loss
For Teens

Joanne Ikeda, MA, RD

Bull Publishing Company

PALO ALTO, CA

Cover Design: Cherlyn Oto
Cover Photo: Steven Oto
Teens in Cover Photo: (left to right)
Zack Reiheld, Sarah Newcomb, Elizabeth Hurst.
Interior Design: Maura McAndrew

ISBN 0-915950-84-7
Printed in the United States

Bull Publishing Company
P.O. Box 208
Palo Alto, CA 94302-0208
(415) 322-2855

Distributed in the United States by:
Publishers Group West
5855 Beaudry Street
Emeryville, CA 94608

Library of Congress Cataloging-in-Publication Data

Ikeda, Joanne P.
    Winning weight loss for teens.

Summary: Presents a program to change poor eating
habits, designed to help young people lose weight and
keep it off.
    1. Children—Nutrition.   2. Reducing diets.
3. Reducing—Psychological aspects.   [1. Weight control.
2. Diet]   I. Title.
RJ206.I27   1987   613.2'5'024055   87-12962
ISBN 0-915950-84-7

Contents

Dedicated with sincere appreciation and love
TO JOAN WONG,
my daughters' second mother.

DEAR TEENAGER,

This is a book for teen-agers that will provide you with a program that you can adapt to your personal situation. You can make it unique to suit your personal needs.

But as a teen-ager, you do not live alone. You probably still live at home — and your parents are a major force in your life. As such, they can hurt or help you in your weight control program.

There are some specific challenges that you face in trying to control your weight that are not always obvious to parents. It will help you if your parents learn about them. So I have tried to cover some of the most important points in the letter to parents that begins on the next page.

If you, the teen-ager who uses this book, share the letter with your parent, it might help that parent to help you. And it will help you to understand the support they can give.

SINCERELY,

Joanne Ikeda

DEAR PARENT,

I write this letter both as a parent and as a nutritionist who has worked with many overweight teenagers. My hope is that I can give you some insight into how you can best help your youngster.

If I could give you only one piece of advice, it would be to urge you to reassure your youngster as often as possible, and in as many ways as possible that s/he is a lovable and worthwhile human being. Most of the youngsters I have worked with have been very worried about their weight. They know that our society discriminates against fat people in many subtle and also not-so-subtle ways. They are frightened that they might end up being unloved and unwanted as well as fat. You need to let your child know that this is not going to happen — s/he will always be loved by you no matter how fat or thin the body.

Recognize your child's positive attributes, and let your child know that you're proud of them. Build up your child's self-confidence and self-esteem to the point where s/he isn't afraid that overweight means rejection and failure.

Putting pressure on a youngster to lose weight, even when it's couched in supportive and helpful terms, may end up being counter-productive. The message the child thinks s/he hears is, "There is something wrong with me, namely that I'm too fat. You would love me more if I was thinner."

Youngsters react to this in a variety of ways. Some get angry and rebellious: "Who do they think they are? I'll eat as much as I want whenever I want." Some get depressed: "They're right, I'm going to end up being a fat slob. No one will want to be my friend or date me except another fat slob." Almost all youngsters lose some self-esteem: "There must be something wrong with me, otherwise I wouldn't be fat. If I was a better person, I would be thinner."

So how can you be helpful and supportive without your child feeling pressured? Actually, there are a number of things you can do. The one highest on my list is to encourage your child to become more physically active. The newest research findings show that many overweight youngsters eat about the same amount of food as normal-weight youngsters. In order to lose weight, they will need to reduce their calorie intake to some extent (and there are lots of suggestions in the book on how to manage overeating), but it is also critical that they use up calories by increasing physical activity. Your child will need to spend more time walking, running, swimming, dancing and so on than ever before.

You can be supportive by offering to join your child in some regular daily activity, such as taking a walk together after dinner every night, or riding bikes together early in the morning before school and work. Your youngster may also need your help in getting to places where s/he can participate in physical activity. You may need to join a car pool for the local soccer team, or maybe you can identify a bus route your child can take to get to the nearest swimming pool.

Your youngster may want to participate in some activity that costs money. You'll need to decide whether you can afford to subsidize aerobic dance classes, tennis lessons, and the like. The local "Y" or city parks and recreation departments often sponsor inexpensive classes.

All parents have limited time, energy, and money, so don't feel you have to provide everything. Select what fits your family lifestyle and resources. One thing for sure, you'll be using your resource on a most important investment for the future — your child.

I'd also like to advise you to be alert for desperation measures on the part of your child to lose weight. Some teenagers go on a lengthy fast and literally starve themselves in order to lose weight. Others adopt abusive practices like self–induced vomiting or overuse of laxatives. Such practices are not just unhealthy — they can be life threatening!

Don't delay talking to your child about your concern. The earlier your child receives help in dealing with such behaviors before they become habits, the better. The research literature documents that people who resort to desperation measures to lose weight only become unhealthy and unhappy, and usually end up needing prolonged professional treatment for eating disorders.

And now for the nutrition advice! My experience leads me to believe that most Americans know that a healthy diet is composed of a variety of foods from the basic food groups, that are low in sodium, sugar, and fat, and are high in complex carbohydrates and fiber. (For this basic nutrition information, send for the free booklet put out by the U.S. Government; write: "Dietary Guidelines for Americans," Consumer Information, Pueblo, Colorado, 81009.) The hard part comes in actually making changes to conform to this ideal.

Here are some suggestions for initiating changes in the family diet:

1. *Identify the major problem(s) with your present family diet (check the problem(s) you are most concerned about).*

   Our diet is _____ *Too high in fat*

   _____ *Too high in sodium*

   _____ *Too high in sugar*

   _____ *Too low in complex carbohydrates*

   _____ *Too low in fiber*

2. *List all the ways you could change your diet in order to correct the problem(s). For example, if your diet is too high in fat, you might list these possible ways to change it:*

   ▶ *Bake, broil, or boil rather than fry food.*

   ▶ *Choose fruit more often for snacks — cut down on corn chips, potato chips and ice cream.*

   ▶ *Drink low-fat or nonfat milk rather than whole milk.*

   ▶ *Trim all visible fat from meat.*

   ▶ *Eat fish and poultry more often.*

   ▶ *Remove the skin from poultry before cooking.*

   ▶ *Don't eat french fries at fast food restaurants.*

3. *Review the list you have made. Cross out any changes that you think everyone in your family will reject. If your family eats at fast-food restaurants only once or twice a month, leaving french fries off the menu won't help that much, especially if you still choose a lot of their other high-fat foods (e.g., hamburgers, shakes, cheeseburgers, onion rings), and it may not be worth the unhappiness it might cause.*

   On the other hand, switching to more fruit for snacks may be very acceptable to your family. Most of them probably like fruit, and they would choose it more often if there was a wider variety available, and if the chips and ice cream weren't there.

Try to end up with at least 4 ways in which you want to change your diet for the better after you're through reviewing your list.

4. *Explain your plan to other family members and invite their input. They may decide to put some of the "rejects" back on the list, or vice versa. It also gets them used to the idea that everyone in the family is going to be making some dietary changes for the better.*

5. *Implement the changes one at a time, leaving at least two weeks between each new change. Many people make the mistake of trying to make too many changes at once. They find that they are not succeeding, so they give up. It is much better to go slowly and be successful.*

These dietary changes will benefit the entire family. Your overweight child will be part of a group effort, where everyone is trying to change his or her diet for the better, not just the one with a weight problem. Overweight youngsters often have a difficult time when they are the only one singled out to make diet and activity changes. When everyone gets in on the act, the mutual support gives far greater promise of success.

Finally, do not burden yourself with guilt about the fact that your child is overweight. If you feel guilty, depressed, and have a poor opinion of yourself, you won't be able to help your child handle these same kinds of feelings. The two of you will only reinforce them in each other!

If you feel good about yourself as a parent, it will be much easier for you to feel good about your child. And that, as I said at the beginning, is how you can best help your overweight child.

SINCERELY,

1

I Want To Lose Weight

I want to look good — to myself and others.

It's natural to want to look good. In America, most people who are considered attractive are slender. This makes sense from a health standpoint. Slim people tend to live longer. They are less apt to suffer from diabetes and coronary heart disease. This leads into the next reason for losing weight.

I want to feel good.

Do you like to backpack, bicycle, dance? Doing anything that's fun means being able to move around easily. When you're fat, you tend to be lazier because moving around is more tiring than when you're trimmer. As you lose weight, you'll find you have more energy to do things.

OK, I've tried before,
what's different about this time?

You've probably tried to lose weight by going on a "diet." The diet advised you to eat certain foods and to avoid other foods.

This was probably harder than it sounds because the diet may not have included many foods you liked. After awhile, you got tired of the diet, or it didn't seem to be doing you any good, so you quit. Maybe you even lost weight on the diet, but afterwards, you put the weight right back on. In any case, you tried to solve your weight problem by temporarily changing the food you were eating.

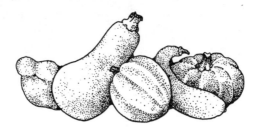

This time you are not going to go on a diet. Instead, you are going to go to the root of your fat problem — bad food and activity habits. You are going to find out which habits are leading you down the path to overweight. Then you are going to think of some creative ways to get off that path and on to the one heading towards a skinnier you!

I'm not going to go on a diet!!

No, you're not going to go on a diet. You're going to try a better way. It's the most successful approach to losing weight and keeping weight off that has ever been tried. Instead of changing the food you eat, you are going to change your eating and activity habits.

Eating habits are things like the time of day you eat, where you eat, how fast you eat, and the "signals" that unconsciously tell you to eat. Activity habits describe how physically active you are. Are you a "walker" or a "rider," a "sitter" or a "stander," a "doer" or a "watcher"?

Sound interesting? It is! And it's fun too. You'll be learning a lot about yourself.

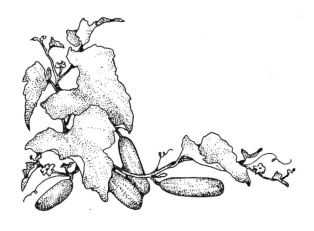

I need a friend.

I'll ask _____ *to help me.*

Face it, you can't do it alone. That doesn't make you unusual or weak-willed. It means you're a member of the human race. A friend can help you in so many ways. S/he can remind you of your commitment to losing weight. S/he can point out ways you can change your habits. Losing can become a game and a challenge rather than a punishment.

Most of all a good friend can reward you with compliments and encouragement. Pick someone you like who likes you. It should be someone you see fairly often, at least two or three times a week, and maybe every day. Perhaps your friend is overweight and wants to join you in losing. Fine, but don't push. The desire to lose can't be borrowed. It has to come from within. That's why it's important for you to believe you can do it!

I'd like to lose _____ *pounds in* _____ *months.*

Would you like to lose 5 pounds, 10, 15, maybe 20? Decide how much you want to lose in the next 3 to 6 months. Frankly, if you try to lose 10 pounds in a month, you're going to get depressed and discouraged. You might even give up, because it's just too hard to lose that much weight in such a short time. You would have to eat so little food, or exercise so much, that you would be hungry, tired and exhausted all the time. A realistic goal is 1 to 2 pounds a week. That means you can eat enough food so you're not starving all the time, but you can still cut down enough to lose weight.

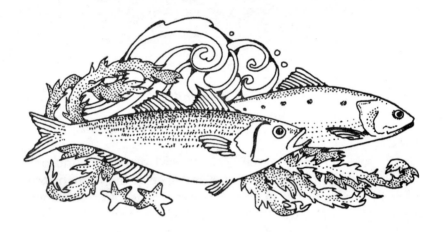

While I lose, I'll gain.

Yes, you'll lose weight, but you're going to gain something too. A better nourished, healthier you! As you improve your diet and become more active, you are going to feel and look better. Your body will be in better shape. You are going to provide it with all of the basic nutrients that it needs, like protein, vitamins, and minerals. Plus you will exercise it to the point where there is less fat in your body and more lean muscle.

Even if your weight plateaus for a while and you don't lose, you'll find yourself looking and feeling better. Your skin will be more elastic and less baggy. Your shape will change. Instead of bands of fat, you'll have a firmer, thinner layer of lean tissue underneath your skin. You'll feel more energetic and full of life.

Whenever you get discouraged about losing weight, remember, there are many benefits coming to you because of the changes you are making. Lower numbers on a scale don't tell the whole story of what is happening to you.

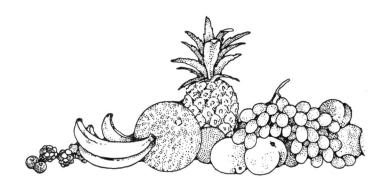

I really mean it.

You've set goals. You have a friend. Now you're ready to make THE commitment. You're going to sign a contract. What! A contract? What does a contract have to do with losing weight?

A whole lot. It says that you mean it — in black and white. It's a commitment you can read over to yourself when the going gets rough. Your friend knows you mean it. S/he saw you sign it. No, it's not silly, so do it.

Here is a sample contract. You can use it, or you can write your own. See Chapter 8 for ideas on rewards.

CONTRACT

KNOW ALL MEN (AND WOMEN) BY THESE PRESENTS:

Whereas and wherefore _____
YOUR NAME

(hereafter called the "loser")

desires to lose _____ pounds in _____ months; and WHEREAS AND
NUMBER NUMBER

WHEREFORE FURTHER, THE UNDERSIGNED FRIEND _____
FRIEND'S NAME

(hereafter called "the friend") promises to assist:

Now therefore, in consideration of the foregoing, the undersigned "friend"
agrees to:

1. **Read the food and activity diary over with "the loser" to check for habits
   that are leading to overwieght.**
2. **Encourage physical exercise by** _____ **with "the loser" as often as possible.**

   jogging, biking, playing badminton...

3. **Not tempt "the loser" to eat.**

4. Offer compliments and support when "the loser" sticks to his/her plans for change. Not comment otherwise.
5. Reward "the loser" by _____

"The loser" has set the following conditions so that s/he will lose weight:

1. I will keep a food and activity diary for at least two weeks, so I can pinpoint the habits I need to change.
2. I will outline plans for changing my habits slowly over time, and I will do my best to stick to these plans.
3. I will outline plans for getting more exercise, and I will do my best to stick to these plans.
4. I will not weigh myself every day or even every week. I realize that the scale is not an accurate way to measure my success. I will judge my success by how well I am doing at changing my food habits.

Neither party will tease, nag or heckle the other. This contract and all information associated with it is to be keep confidential unless otherwise noted.

_____
("THE LOSERS" SIGNATURE)

_____
(DATE)

_____
("THE FRIEND'S" SIGNATURE)

_____
(DATE)

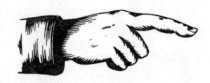

You Are Ready To Go On To Chapter Two
IF:

_____ You have a friend who will give you support and encouragement.

_____ You signed a contract with your friend.

_____ You set a reasonable weight loss goal.

_____ You recognize all the benefits of changing your food and activity patterns.

_____ You believe that you can do it!

2

The Food Diary —
My Most Important Tool
For Losing Weight

*"Dear diary, at 3 pm today while walking home
with Meg, I ate 16 peanuts and 4 Tootsie Rolls."*

In order to lose weight, you are going to change your food
habits. But, maybe some of your food habits are pretty good!
Maybe you don't need to change them. On the other hand,
you've got some food habits that aren't so good — the ones
that are making you overweight. How can you tell the good
habits from the bad ones? How do you even know what your
habits are — good and bad?

That's a real problem — you don't. But you can find out.
The way to do it is to keep a food diary.

Your food diary is your most important tool for losing
weight. It may be a drag to keep, but you'll be glad you're
doing it once you see how useful it is to you.

First, it will help you cut down on the amount of food you
eat. Every time you eat and then write in the food diary, it
will remind you of everything else you've **eaten that day.**

9

Secondly, the food diary will help you see the food habits that are causing your weight problem.

After you've kept the food diary for two weeks, sit down and look it over very closely. Try to find trends in your eating — things you find you're doing over and over again. Use the sheets in this book — you can fold them up and keep them in your pocket or purse.

The rest of this chapter will guide you in examining your food diary. But the first step is to start keeping it. So now is the time!

► **The times of day you eat**

Write down the time of day you eat, every time you eat.

► **The number of minutes you spend eating**

Notice the time you start eating and the time you finish. Write in your diary the number of minutes you spend eating.

► **The place where you're eating**

Notice where you are when you eat...in the kitchen...at the school snack bar...in your bedroom.

► **Your other activities while eating**

Write down what else you're doing while you're eating, such as watching TV or talking on the telephone.

► **How hungry you feel when you begin eating**

Rate your hunger on a scale of 1 to 4.
1 = full, 2 = not full, but not hungry,
3 = hungry, 4 = starved!

► **Your mood**

What mood are you in each time you eat? Happy? Sad? Mad? Worried? Bored?

► **The food and the amount you eat**

Keep an accurate record of the foods you eat and the amount you eat. Most people are not very good at judging amounts. You may want to try measuring your helpings at home for the first week.

► **Calories**

The number of calories in the foods you are eating. This is an "optional" column. If you already know which foods are high in calories, and which are low, you don't really need to fill in this column. But, if you don't know that much about calories, pick up some basic facts by reading Chapter 5 on "Just Give Me the Facts." Then buy an inexpensive calorie booklet at a local bookstore. Look up the foods you are eating in the calorie booklet and keep track of them by filling in the calorie column.

You will need to keep the food diary for at least 2 weeks. This will give you an accurate picture of your current food habits. You may even decide to continue keeping the food diary all during your efforts to lose weight. This is a smart move — you'll get lots of feedback from it.

It's all right to go on and read the rest of this book while keeping the food diary, but don't try to keep other records or make changes until after keeping the diary for two weeks.

Start keeping your food diary today! There is no reason to delay. Keep it for the next two weeks. Then for help on analyzing your food diary, read Chapter Three.

NOTE: You will find additional Food Diary forms at the back of the book. Feel free to photocopy for additional copies as you need them.

FOOD DIARY

Day April 26th

Time of Day	Minutes Spent Eating	Places You Eat	Other Activity While Eating	How Hungry You Feel	Mood	Food	Amount	Calories
noon	15	School Yard	Talking with friends	HUNGRY – No Breakfast –3	Feeling Good	Tuna Sandwich	2 slice bread ¼ cup tuna 1 Tbsp. Mayo	140 150 100
						Chocolate Milk (low-fat)	8 oz Glass	190
						Banana	1 Medium	110

FOOD DIARY

Day ___

Time of Day	Minutes Spent Eating	Places You Eat	Other Activity While Eating	How Hungry You Feel	Mood	Food	Amount	Calories

FOOD DIARY

Day _____

Time of Day	Minutes Spent Eating	Places You Eat	Other Activity While Eating	How Hungry You Feel	Mood	Food	Amount	Calories

FOOD DIARY

Day _____

Time of Day	Minutes Spent Eating	Places You Eat	Other Activity While Eating	How Hungry You Feel	Mood	Food	Amount	Calories

FOOD DIARY

Day _____

Time of Day	Minutes Spent Eating	Places You Eat	Other Activity While Eating	How Hungry You Feel	Mood	Food	Amount	Calories

13a

FOOD DIARY

Day _____

Time of Day	Minutes Spent Eating	Places You Eat	Other Activity While Eating	How Hungry You Feel	Mood	Food	Amount	Calories

FOOD DIARY

Day _____

Time of Day	Minutes Spent Eating	Places You Eat	Other Activity While Eating	How Hungry You Feel	Mood	Food	Amount	Calories

14a

FOOD DIARY

Day _____

Time of Day	Minutes Spent Eating	Places You Eat	Other Activity While Eating	How Hungry You Feel	Mood	Food	Amount	Calories

FOOD DIARY

Day ___

Time of Day	Minutes Spent Eating	Places You Eat	Other Activity While Eating	How Hungry You Feel	Mood	Food	Amount	Calories

FOOD DIARY

Day _____

Time of Day	Minutes Spent Eating	Places You Eat	Other Activity While Eating	How Hungry You Feel	Mood	Food	Amount	Calories

16

FOOD DIARY

Day ____

Time of Day	Minutes Spent Eating	Places You Eat	Other Activity While Eating	How Hungry You Feel	Mood	Food	Amount	Calories

16a

FOOD DIARY

Day ____

Time of Day	Minutes Spent Eating	Places You Eat	Other Activity While Eating	How Hungry You Feel	Mood	Food	Amount	Calories

FOOD DIARY

Day ___

Time of Day	Minutes Spent Eating	Places You Eat	Other Activity While Eating	How Hungry You Feel	Mood	Food	Amount	Calories

FOOD DIARY

Day _____

Time of Day	Minutes Spent Eating	Places You Eat	Other Activity While Eating	How Hungry You Feel	Mood	Food	Amount	Calories

FOOD DIARY

Day _____

Time of Day	Minutes Spent Eating	Places You Eat	Other Activity While Eating	How Hungry You Feel	Mood	Food	Amount	Calories

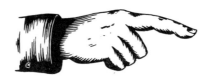

You Are Ready To Go On To Chapter Three
IF:

_____ You have filled in the Food Diary every
day for 14 days. (If you have only filled
it in intermittently, try to keep it for at
least 6 days in a row before going on
to the next chapter.)

~3~

Use Your Food Diary
To Learn About Yourself

Give it a careful going over.

Now that you have kept your food diary for two weeks, you are ready to look it over carefully. You are going to take time to look at each of the categories (such as "Time," "Minutes Spent Eating," "Other Activity While Eating," etc.). The next sections in this chapter will tell you what to look for under each category. There will be suggestions about what to do, depending on what you find you have written down.

Before filling in any forms in this chapter, read ahead up to and including the section on Setting Priorities on page 35. Then keep in mind as you fill in the following forms that you will eventually decide what your priorities are for putting them into action.

I don't eat breakfast or lunch, I'm on a diet!

Check the "Time" category for each day you filled in the food diary. Are you eating about the same number of meals and

snacks around the same times every day? Or, do you
have irregular eating habits — sometimes you eat at 10 AM
and 3 PM, other times you start eating at 11:30 AM? It is
very important to try to establish more regular eating
patterns. Then you'll be in better control of your eating.

Eventually you will want to eat 3 meals and 2 snacks a day.
Of course, these won't be huge meals and high-calorie snacks,
but there will be foods you like! (See Chapter 4 for advice on
calories and servings.) Studies of people who have been
successful at losing weight (compared to people who haven't
been successful) show that the successful people tended to
eat at least 3 and up to 6 times a day! The people who were
unsuccessful dieters and didn't lose weight, never ate breakfast, rarely ate lunch, and usually nibbled most of the evening
hours.

In the long run, the people who ate regular meals and
snacks ended up eating fewer calories than those who ate
only twice a day. The people who skipped meals because
they were "dieting" were so starved by the end of the day
that they binged on huge amounts of food. Those who didn't
skip meals weren't hungry all the time and weren't tempted
to overeat. So your first step is to try gradually to adopt more
regular meal patterns.

If you have irregular eating habits and you want to do
something about them, try to change gradually. Don't decide
that next week you're going to eat breakfast every day and
never skip lunch. That's unrealistic and you won't stick to
it. You're setting too high a goal for yourself. Be easy on

yourself, instead; say, "Next week I'll eat a 'carry-along' breakfast two days, and if I manage that, the following week I'll eat breakfast three days."

Set a small, reachable goal for yourself. Your "carry-along" breakfast might be an orange and a cheese slice melted on whole wheat bread. It could be an apple and carton of low-fat yogurt. If you've got a few minutes at home, heat up a small frozen pizza and have it with a glass of orange juice. Pour a bowl of cereal and add low-fat milk. Breakfast doesn't have to be bacon and eggs or pancakes and sausage, even though these are traditional breakfast foods. There's no rule that says you have to eat these foods in the morning.

Increase the number of regular meals only when you've been successful the previous week. If you planned to eat breakfast twice in the last week but didn't, then don't plan on eating breakfast three times next week. See if you can get to two breakfasts before you try for three. The same goes for lunch. If you're only eating lunch three times a week, try to increase it to four times. Once you've made it to four, try five. Eventually you should work up to a point where you are eating three meals a day most days.

My plans for change.

Right now I eat breakfast _____ times a week. Next week, I'm going to try to eat breakfast _____ times. If I'm successful at doing that, the following week I'll try to eat breakfast _____ mornings. I think I'll be doing well if I gradually work up to eating breakfast _____ times each week.

Keep Score.

Write a "B" on each day you plan to have breakfast. Draw a star with a red pen over the "B" if you do eat breakfast on that day.

WEEK #1

Monday	Tuesday	Wednesday	Thursday	Friday	Saturday	Sunday

WEEK #2

Monday	Tuesday	Wednesday	Thursday	Friday	Saturday	Sunday

WEEK #3

Monday	Tuesday	Wednesday	Thursday	Friday	Saturday	Sunday

WEEK #4

Monday	Tuesday	Wednesday	Thursday	Friday	Saturday	Sunday

My plans for change.

Right now I eat lunch _____ times a week. Next week I'm going to try to eat lunch _____ times. If I'm successful at doing that, the following week I'll try to eat lunch _____ times. I think I'll be doing well if I gradually work up to eating lunch _____ times a week.

Keep Score.

Write an "L" on each day you plan to eat lunch. Draw a star with a red pen over the "L" if you do eat lunch on that day.

WEEK #1

Monday	Tuesday	Wednesday	Thursday	Friday	Saturday	Sunday

WEEK #2

Monday	Tuesday	Wednesday	Thursday	Friday	Saturday	Sunday

WEEK #3

Monday	Tuesday	Wednesday	Thursday	Friday	Saturday	Sunday

WEEK #4

Monday	Tuesday	Wednesday	Thursday	Friday	Saturday	Sunday

I'm always through eating before everyone else.

Check the column in your food diary listing the number of "Minutes Spent Eating." Are you taking 10 minutes to eat a whole meal and gulping down a snack in a minute or two? Whoa there! Time to slow down your eating. Time to enjoy the taste sensations in your mouth. Here are some simple ways to do it:

▶ Lay your spoon or fork down between each bite of food.

► Try chewing your food more slowly. You may want to count how many times you chew each mouthful before you swallow. Then try to increase the number of chews you make before swallowing.

► Take a sip of water between every other bite of food.

► Think about the flavors you can taste in each bite.

► If you're eating with someone else, talk about something pleasant (but not with food in your mouth!).

My plans for change.

I take about _____ minutes to eat most meals. I'd like to increase my eating time to about _____ minutes per meal. I'm going to try to do this by _____

Keep Score.

Write "slow down" next to the meals you are going to practice eating more slowly. Draw a star with a red pen over the "slow down" when you do take longer to eat at these meals.

WEEK #1

	Monday	Tuesday	Wednesday	Thursday	Friday	Saturday	Sunday
Breakfast							
Lunch							
Dinner							

WEEK #2

	Monday	Tuesday	Wednesday	Thursday	Friday	Saturday	Sunday
Breakfast							
Lunch							
Dinner							

WEEK #3

	Monday	Tuesday	Wednesday	Thursday	Friday	Saturday	Sunday
Breakfast							
Lunch							
Dinner							

WEEK #4

	Monday	Tuesday	Wednesday	Thursday	Friday	Saturday	Sunday
Breakfast							
Lunch							
Dinner							

*I eat in my bedroom, in the living room,
in the kitchen, at the school snack bar...*

Look over the "Places You Eat" column in the food diary. Where are you doing most of your eating? What locations say "EAT" to your unconscious mind? Maybe there are a lot of them — your bedroom, the living room, the kitchen. Every time you're in these rooms you feel like eating. How can you change this? One way is to choose a spot in your home to do all of your eating. The most likely location is a kitchen or dining area table, but it doesn't have to be there. It's your choice. Make this eating area as attractive as possible. Have a pretty placemat, some colored napkins, a nice mug.

Then always sit in this same place whenever you eat anything at home...even if it's just a bunch of grapes. After awhile you'll find the other rooms in the house won't trigger eating. You won't be nearly as tempted to snack in those places as you had been! This will be especially true if you don't keep food in easy reach. Out go the box of crackers under your bed and the dish of candy in the living room! Even in the kitchen, it will help to keep food behind cupboard doors. Why tempt yourself?

My plans for change.

I eat a lot in the _____
When I'm at home, I'll eat only in the_____
I need to remove food from the following places so it won't be there to tempt me: _____

Keep Score.

Draw a star with a red pen on each day you keep your resolution to eat only in one location in your home.

	Monday	Tuesday	Wednesday	Thursday	Friday	Saturday	Sunday
Week #1							
Week #2							
Week #3							
Week #4							

Gee, do I always eat while I'm watching TV?

Do you eat while you watch TV, study, talk on the telephone? Check the "Other Activity While Eating" column of your food diary to find out. Just as certain locations can trigger eating, so can activities. If you find that you often eat while doing something else, you may want to try to break this association. For example, one person who didn't think she overate much looked at her food diary and discovered that she constantly nibbled while talking on the phone to friends. She realized that if she wanted to lose weight, she needed to change this habit.

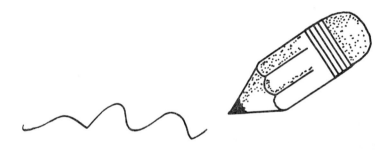

One way to do it was mentioned in the last section — choosing a specific place in your house to do all of your eating. Another idea is to keep your hands busy so you don't feel tempted to reach for food. Try working on a jigsaw puzzle or doodling with a pencil or writing and underlining key words. Keep food out of reach so it won't be so handy to start nibbling.

My plans for change.

I eat a lot when I'm_____
I think I can stop doing this if I_____
_____

Keep Score.

Write an "E" on each day you plan to practice eating without any accompanying activities. Draw a star with a red pen over the "E" on days you accomplish this goal.

	Monday	Tuesday	Wednesday	Thursday	Friday	Saturday	Sunday
Week #1							
Week #2							
Week #3							
Week #4							

I'm hungry all the time.

Looking over the "How Hungry You Feel" column, did you find that you really were hungry every time you ate? Probably not. We're often tempted to eat by other things — friends who want us to stop for a snack, the smell of food as we walk by a bakery or restaurant, or the sight of food on a TV commercial or a sign. Before you eat, ask youself, am I really hungry? Do I really want to eat now or should I wait until later when I'm hungry?

What if you are hungry a lot of the time? How can you deal with your hunger pangs? Here are some suggestions:

▶ Wait 15 to 20 minutes before eating. Hunger pangs usually don't last for more than 10 to 15 minutes. If you delay eating, your hunger may go away and you won't eat after all.

▶ Drink a half glass of orange, apple or grapefruit juice, or hot tea or boullion. Juice or a hot drink will usually help hunger pangs to disappear.

► Become involved in some other activity so you won't think about how hungry you feel. Think of two or three activities that will take your mind off eating. Get so involved in them that you forget you are hungry.

My plans for change.

When I feel hungry, I'll _____ instead of eating right away.

Keep Score.

Write a capital "H" on each day you plan not to eat every time you feel hungry. Draw a star with a red pen over the "H" on days you accomplish this.

	Monday	Tuesday	Wednesday	Thursday	Friday	Saturday	Sunday
Week #1							
Week #2							
Week #3							
Week #4							

I really deserve a hot fudge sundae.

Look at the "Mood" column in your food diary. Are certain moods stimulating you to eat? Do you eat to reward yourself? (You passed the math exam and you really deserve a "treat.") Maybe you eat to console yourself? (It's been a rough week and that special person didn't call after all, so why not drown yourself in chocolate ice cream.)

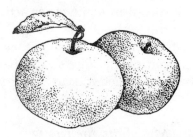

It's not unusual to use food in these ways. After all, didn't your mom buy you an ice cream cone when you were good on the shopping trip? Didn't she give you a cookie and a hug when you came home crying after you fell off your bike? We've been taught to use food to reward and console ourselves, and it's hard to break the habit.

It may be impossible to completely avoid using food for emotional reasons, but it's a good idea to try to minimize it. You can do that by thinking of other ways to reward and console yourself (see Chapter 8). If you find that you are often depressed, you may want to talk to a professional counselor. Check with your school counselor or the local mental health association for a referral. If you are occasionally depressed, you can use "positive thoughts" to counter these low moods. Here are some suggestions:

> ► Think of 5 things you really like about your-self. Maybe you are good at fixing things. Perhaps you have long graceful fingers. Don't start off on a negative trip, saying "I'm short and dumpy; I'll never be good looking." Concentrate on the positive.

5 things I like about me.

1. _____

2. _____

3. _____

4. _____

5. _____

► What turns you on? Christmas tree lights? The warmth of your house after walking home from school on a cold day? Make a list of 10 things in your life that make you feel good. When you get depressed, add 2 or 3 more things to the list. Read the list over and try to experience each of these things in your mind's eye.

I feel good when I...

1. _____
2. _____
3. _____
4. _____
5. _____
6. _____
7. _____
8. _____
9. _____
10. _____

Did I really eat that much food yesterday?

The food diary columns for, "Food" and "Amount" are your record of how much you eat each day. You'll probably find you eat less than usual once you start keeping the food diary. This is because each time you write in the diary you can see all the other times you've eaten, and you may decide to forgo the next snack. Most people who keep food diaries discover they automatically cut their food intake about 10%. This is the reason it isn't necessary to stick to a rigid calorie-restricted diet in order to lose weight.

This column can also help you evaluate the kind of food you are eating in terms of nutrition, calories, and serving sizes. See Chapter 5 for pointers.

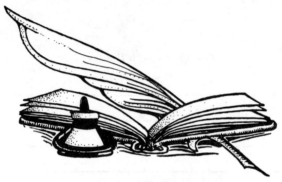

I'm learning about me!

Surprised at some of the things you found out about yourself by keeping the food diary? You probably didn't realize you had many of these habits, and you never would have found out if you didn't keep the food diary. It is an essential tool for losing weight.

Now that you've pinpointed some of your problems, you're ready to begin changing some of your habits. But, you need to decide what to work on first. Do you want to slow down your eating at meal time? Would you like to try eating at only one spot in your house? Maybe you're convinced you need to adopt more regular meal patterns? Or, do you want to do all of those things right now?

Setting Priorities

STOP! Don't be unrealistic. It's hard to change. If you try to make too many changes at one time, you won't succeed at any of them and you might even be tempted to quit! Instead, set some priorities. Ask yourself what the major problems are and begin to work on those first. Here is a list of potential changes you might want to make. Check the ones you think you need to make, based on the information in your food diary. Then, number the ones you've checked according to the order in which you're going to work on them.

CHANGES I NEED TO MAKE	CHANGES NUMBERED IN ORDER OF PRIORITY	CHANGES
_____	_____	I need to start eating in the morning.
_____	_____	I need to start eating lunch more frequently.
_____	_____	I need to slow down my eating.
_____	_____	I need to eat in one spot in the house.
_____	_____	I need to get rid of foods that are tempting me to overeat.
_____	_____	I need to learn to eat without any accompanying activity.
_____	_____	I need to deal with my constant hunger.
_____	_____	I need to stop using food to reward or console myself.

I want it to happen fast.

It will take you 3 to 6 months to change your food habits and to reach your weight loss goal. If this seems like a long time, remember, you spent a lifetime developing these habits and it's only natural to take awhile to change them. Keep track of your success by using the calendars provided in the different sections. The more red stars on your calendars, the better your chances are for losing weight. If you find that one kind of change is not working for you, go on to another. But try not to skip around too much. Give each change a real chance before giving up and going on to something else.

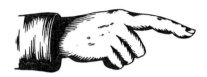

You Are Ready To Go On To Chapter Four
IF:

_____ You've looked over the food diary carefully and pinpointed the food habits you want to change.

_____ You have decided the order in which you are going to try to make these changes.

_____ You are using the calendars and red stars to keep track of your program.

4

What Do I Do To Lose Weight Besides Diet?

I've got the answer.

What else can you do to lose weight besides diet? You probably know the answer. In order to lose weight you should eat fewer calories **and you should become more physically active.**

For total fitness, nothing beats aerobics.

Aerobic exercise — sounds pretty sophisticated doesn't it? It's actually basic to your physical fitness. Aerobic exercise is exercise that makes your heart beat faster for a sustained period of time, by increasing the body's need for oxygen. This type of exercise benefits the entire body, by strengthening the heart, lungs, and circulatory system. It also increases the amount of lean body mass and decreases the amount of fat in your body.

Jogging, running, brisk walking, rowing, jumping rope, swimming, skiing, cycling, aerobic dancing, skating, hiking (uphill), and playing tennis, racquetball, basketball, soccer, squash, and handball can be effective aerobic exercises, if they are done briskly for at least 30 minutes at least 3 times a week. If you are serious about losing weight and becoming physically fit, aerobic exercise needs to become a part of your life.

But wait! Don't jump right in and begin! Always spend at least 5 minutes doing stretching exercises to "warm-up" before you start any aerobic exercise. These exercises will stretch the muscles and prepare the joints for moving through a range of motions. They give the body a chance to get ready for vigorous exercise. For stretching warm-up exercises, see the section in this chapter on "I'd like my waist to waste away."

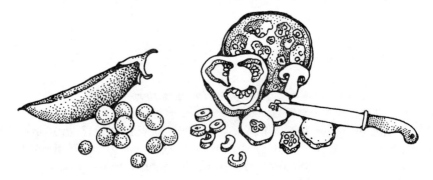

Build up the time you spend on aerobic exercise gradually. The first time you try it, aim for 15 minutes, plus a 5-minute warm-up and a 5-minute cool-down (see p. 48). Add on 5 more minutes of aerobics the next time, and another 5 minutes every time until you reach your goal level. Always begin and end with the 5-minute warm-up and the 5-minute cool-down periods.

If you try to be superperson, and exercise vigorously for too long the first few times you exercise, you can easily end up hurting yourself; so listen to people in the know and build up your level of activity gradually.

For the 5-minute cool-down after you have finished aerobic exercising, use the same exercises you used to warm-up. This will prevent your muscles from becoming sore, and allow your circulatory system to return to normal without cramping.

MY AEROBICS CALENDAR

	Monday	Tuesday	Wednesday	Thursday	Friday	Saturday	Sunday
Week #1							
Week #2							
Week #3							

Keep track.

Write in the kind of aerobic exercise, and the time spent each day for the next three weeks, or until it is a regular part of your routine.

But I'm no athlete.

Does the thought of exercising depress you? Are you re-membering the way you look in shorts and thinking how ridiculous you feel on the field or court? Do people yell at you to "Get that ball!" — when you know there is no way you are going to get it? Do you cringe at the very idea of organized sports?

Well, stop now and cheer up! You don't have to go out for tennis, basketball, baseball, volleyball, or any other kind of ball unless you yourself want to. There are other options. For instance, in the next chapter you will calculate how much weight you can lose by riding your bike for 30 minutes each day. That's one idea. Here are some others.

1. For at least a half hour each day, put on some records or a videotape and do aerobic dance. (If you have a VCR, buy or borrow a good aerobic exercise tape.) You can lose close to half a pound a week. So shake it up!

2. Swim for a half hour two or three times a week. You don't have a pool? The local park and recreation department, YMCA or YWCA have pools you can use. Check them out.

3. Take a brisk walk after you get home from school, or after finishing your homework (instead of watching TV). There is a direct correlation between TV viewing and overweight! Make sure your prime time isn't spent in front of the set.

4. If you're lucky enough to belong to a health spa or club, use the rowing machine or stationary bicycle. But don't bother with the machines that just jiggle your body around. Massaging fat doesn't reduce it or firm it up; you've got to do the jiggling yourself to accomplish that!

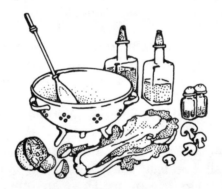

Every day in every way
I'm going to move around more!

There are small things you can do to use up calories. True, in the short run, they won't make much difference in your weight. But, and that's a big BUT, in the long run they can make a real difference. Say you have the choice of riding the bus home from school or taking 20 minutes to walk home. If you walk home, you can lose about 8 pounds in one year.

Even if you ride the bus every other night and walk home half the time, you can still lose 4 pounds. Here are some other suggestions. Check the ones you're going to do.

Moving it more.

_____ I will answer the telephone extension farthest from where I am.

_____ I will stand up while talking on the telephone.

_____ I will use the rest room or bathroom farthest away from me.

_____ I will park the car at the far end of the parking lot.

_____ I will not drive or ride when I can walk.

_____ I will not use the escalator or elevator when stairs are available.

_____ I won't ask my brother/sister/mother/ father to bring me something that I can get for myself.

How many calories do I use each day?

Figuring out the number of calories you burn each day is a real chore. First, you have to keep track of how you spend every minute during a 24-hour time period. Then you need to calculate the number of calories you expended on all your activities, including sleeping (remember, even though you are lying down at rest during sleep, your body is still operating itself). The table on the following page shows the number of calories you will use up for different activities.

► Sleeping, lying down at rest, watching TV, studying — 1 to 1.5 calories per minute

► Sewing, working on your car, typing, playing a musical instrument, ironing, other similar seated and standing activities — up to 2.5 calories per minute

► Walking 2.5 to 3 miles per hour, shopping, carpentry, golfing, sailing, table tennis, volleyball, washing clothes, bowling — 2.5 to 5 calories per minute

► Walking 3.5 to 4 miles per hour, dancing, bicycling, skiing, stacking boxes, scrubbing floors, tennis — 5 to 7.5 calories per minute

► Swimming, basketball, climbing, football, walking uphill while carrying a load, working with a pickax, chopping wood, jogging — 7.5 to 12 calories per minute

What did you do all day (and night)?

To figure out the number of calories you used up in a 24-hour time span:

1. Write down all of your activities during the 24 hours, including sleep. (Obviously you will have to generalize a bit, and not try to account for every separate minute: Record in terms of quarter or half hours at the least, and the type of activity that best describes how you spent that particular block of time.)

2. Write down the number of minutes you spent
   on each activity. This should add up to a
   total of 24 hours, or 1440 minutes.
3. Multiply the number of minutes you spent
   on an activity by the number of calories used
   per minute by the activity. Use the figures
   from the table on the preceding page.
4. Enter the total number of calories used for
   each activity in the last column. Add all these
   numbers up to get a grand total of the number of calories used in a 24-hour time span.

Activity	Number of minutes spent on activity	×	Number of calories used per minute	=	Total number of calories used for each activity
Example: Watching TV	180 minutes		1.5		270

_____

_____

_____

_____

_____

_____

_____

_____

_____

Activity	Number of minutes spent on activity	×	Number of calories used per minute	=	Total number of calories used for each activity

Grand Total: 1440 minutes

There must be an easier way!

It's a lot of work to keep track of the number of calories you use up. One reason some people want to is to tell if they're increasing their physical activity over time. But, there's an easier way to do that. You can go to a local sporting goods store and buy an instrument called a pedometer. A pedometer measures how far you walk each day. You wear it at your waist hung from a belt. The motion of your leg causes the pedometer to function (so don't put it in your purse or hip pocket.)

First you'll want to wear the pedometer on days you aren't making any effort to become more physically active. This will give you some idea of how far you usually walk. Then on the following days, wear the pedometer and make a serious effort to increase your physical activity. Use some of the ideas suggested earlier in this chapter. Check the pedometer. Did you walk more than usual? Challenge yourself to increase your activity so the pedometer measures more miles each day.

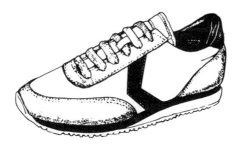

Keep Score.

Write down the number of miles you walk before making any effort to increase your activity level. Then keep track of how many miles you are walking when you are trying to increase your activity.

Before: _____ number of miles walked in one day

	Monday	Tuesday	Wednesday	Thursday	Friday	Saturday	Sunday
Week #1							
Week #2							
Week #3							
Week #4							

I'd like my waist to waste away.

Some people want smaller waists. Others would like slimmer thighs. Still others think their upper arms are too heavy. All want to spot reduce. Many buy gadgets promoted for spot reduction. They attempt to beat, massage, jiggle, or stroke fat away. All to no avail.

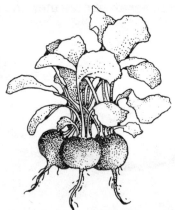

So what can a person do to improve his/her physique? Exercises! Exercising can tone up muscles. Many people who curve out where they should curve in have weak, flabby muscles. Exercise can strengthen these muscles, and really change body measurements. Start out doing a few each day and steadily increase the number.

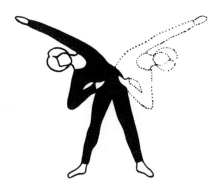

1. WAIST WHITTLER

Position: Stand with legs about 4 inches apart.
Place left hand on hip; raise right arm.

Bend to the left side, slide left hand down leg as
far as possible. Raise body until standing straight
again. Place right hand on hip; raise left arm
overhead. Bend to the right side.

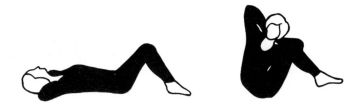

2. BENT-KNEE SIT-UPS
(Strengthens abdominal muscles)

Position: Lie on back with knees bent, hands
clasped behind neck.

Sit up; touch right elbow to left knee. Lie down.
Sit up. Touch left elbow to right knee. Return to
starting position.

* Sketches reprinted courtesy of the Division of Agricultural Sciences,
University of California.

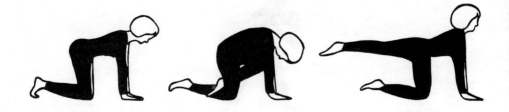

3. KNEE-TO-NOSE TOUCH
(Stretches lower back, strengthens upper back
and hip muscles)

Position: Kneel with hands on floor.
   Try to touch knee to nose and then extend leg
backward, parallel with floor while raising head.
Do not arch back. Switch legs and start again.

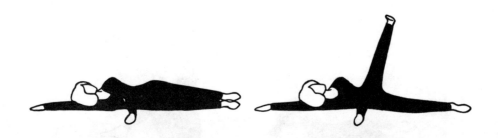

4. SIDE LEG RAISE
(Strengthens muscles on side of hip and thigh)

Position: Lie on side.
   Raise and lower upper leg as high as you can.
Switch sides and start again.

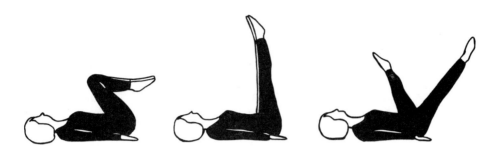

5. LEG SPLITS
(Strengthens muscles on insides of thighs)

Position: Lie on back, raise knees to chest, extend legs until perpendicular to floor.

Slowly lower legs to the sides. Then raise legs until together again. Lower legs slowly to floor. Repeat.

Exercise for odd moments.

Even though you really think it would be a great idea to exercise every day, there are apt to be times when you just don't get around to it. However, there are some exercises you can easily fit into your daily routine that are fun. You do them as you do other things.

RED LIGHT GUT SUCK

While sitting in your car waiting for the light to turn green, suck in your breath and hold in your stomach muscles. Don't breathe or relax your muscles until the light turns green!

TV DEEP KNEE BENDS

Make 3 deep knee bends every time you turn the TV set off or on.

CAR KEY HOP

Hop on one foot as you unlock the car or front door.

BUS STOP JOG

Jog in place while you are waiting for the bus.

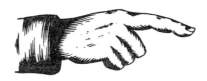

You Are Ready To Go On To Chapter Five
IF:

_____ You have decided on specific ways you are going to become more active.

_____ You are making a daily effort to be more active.

_____ **You are continuing with your plans to change your food habits.**

_____ You are doing aerobic exercise at least 3 times a week, for at least 30 minutes, with a 5 minute warm-up and a 5 minute cool-down period.

5

Just Give Me The Facts

Genetics...Was I born to be fat?

New studies show that genetics does play a role in determining body size. This does not mean that some people are born to be fat and others are born to be thin. However, it does mean that some people are at greater risk of becoming fat than others.

How can you tell if you are at greater risk than average? Look at your closest biological relatives. Are your parents overweight? Are any of your sisters or brothers overweight? If they are, then you are at greater risk than if they were thinner.

Does this doom you to a lifetime of fatness? NO, you are still in control of your destiny. But you will need to be especially careful to control your calorie intake and to exercise regularly throughout your life because your tendency towards fatness will be with you for life.

Ectomorph, mesomorph, or endomorph... weird names for common body builds.

You can blame your ancestors for your body build — there is no question that it is determined by genetics, and inherited.

There are three basic types of body builds. You will fall into one or a combination of these types.

(1) People who have long lean bodies with light skeletons and small muscle development ("ectomorphs"). These people usually don't have overweight problems, but sometimes they are underweight.

(2) People who have large heavy skeletons with lots of muscle development ("mesomorphs"). Mesomorphs may weigh a lot, but at the same time they may not be overfat. The ideal football player is a mesomorph, with a heavy skeleton and lots of developed muscles, but a minimal amount of fat.

(3) People who are round and soft with lots of fat padding their body ("endomorphs"). These people have the most difficult time maintaining normal weight, because their bodies store fat easily.

There is no way you can change your body type. Endomorphs cannot become ectomorphs and vice versa. The thing to do is accept your body build the way it is and make the best of it.

The truth, the whole truth, and nothing but the truth.

The facts about weight control are as follows:

▶ You eat food;

▶ your body uses the food for energy to run itself and for physical activity;

▶ any energy not used for one of these purposes is stored in the body as fat;

▶ if you eat more food energy than your body
  needs to run itself and for physical activity,
  YOU WILL GAIN WEIGHT;

▶ if you eat less food energy than your body
  needs to run itself and for physical activity,
  YOU WILL LOSE WEIGHT.

Another word for food energy is "calories." A calorie is a
measure of energy that food produces. Calories are in food.
All foods with fat, carbohydrate, and protein contain calories.
Vitamins and minerals don't have calories, and neither does
water.

"Calorie" is not a dirty word.

Every BODY needs calories just to stay alive. This food
energy is used by the body to keep the heart beating, the
lungs breathing, the kidneys eliminating waste products, the
cells repairing themselves, new tissues being built, and for
the regulation of body temperature.

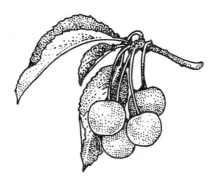

Even when a person is lying quietly or is asleep, s/he still
needs a certain amount of energy to keep the body going.
Scientists refer to this energy as "BMR" or "basal metabolic
rate." It is the amount of energy for basic body processes

necessary for life. The "BMR" ranges from 1300 to 1700 calories, depending on a person's body size, age, sex and secretion of certain hormones. Many people use more calories for body processes they don't control than they use for physical movements they do. Which leads to the second need for calories — for physical activity.

Any time you move your body, you are using up a few calories. It takes some, although not a lot of calories to lift your arm, to move your leg, even to blink your eyes. When you think of physical activity, you probably think of exercise and sports. But physical activity is any time you move. The more you move your body around, the more calories you will use up.

It's not like the good old days.

Have you ever asked your grandparents what their life was like when they were teenagers? Try it. One thing that may surprise you is how much more physically active they were. Maybe not in the sense of sports, but more in terms of their everyday lives. They probably walked to school instead of riding in a car or bus. They had to wash the dishes instead of just loading them into the dishwasher. Your grandmother didn't have a clothes dryer; she hung clothes out on the clothesline to dry. And the clothes weren't "permanent press," they had to be ironed.

Yes, times have changed, and lifestyles have changed too. People are a lot more sedentary. You don't move around as much as your grandparents did. As a result, you need fewer calories than they did when they were your age.

But, food is probably more available to you than it was to them. It's easy to grab a hamburger. The supermarket is filled with tempting snack items to whet your appetite. The TV set constantly bombards you with "EAT" messages. It's harder for you to avoid eating than it was for your grandparents.

In the previous chapters, you learned about ways to increase your physical activity and to escape overeating. This is how physical activity helps you lose weight. Let's say you usually take the bus to and from school each day. Now you decide to ride your bike instead. It takes you about 15 minutes of cycling one way, for a total of 30 minutes of bike riding each day to get to school and back. Figure out how much weight you could lose by doing this for 8 months. (See answer at bottom of page)

30   minutes of bike riding

× 3.5   calories per minute used for bicycling
=   calories used per week

× 7
=   calories used per week

× 32
=   calories used in 8 months (32 weeks)

_____ ÷ ___3,500___ = _____

Number of   Number of   Number of
calories used   calories in   pounds lost
in 8 months   1 pound of fat

How many calories do I need every day?

Do you know how many calories you need every day to maintain your current weight? You can estimate the approximate number by doing some simple multiplication. If you are a girl, multiply your weight by 17. If you are a boy, multiply your current weight by 20.

My current weight is _____ pounds

Multiply by 17 (girl)

20 (boy) _____ calories, approximately, to maintain my current weight.

Warning About Very Low Calorie Diets

Very low calorie diets (under 1200 calories) are dangerous for some people. Anyone considering going on such a diet should consult a physician before doing so, and should be under a doctor's supervision.

But I want to lose weight.

What if you want to lose weight by reducing the number of calories you are eating? There are 3500 in 1 pound of fat. A good weight loss goal to aim for is 1 pound of fat a week. To do this, you must eat 500 calories less each day than your body uses, in order to lose 1 pound in a week. How many calories does this leave you?

_____ Number of calories I need to maintain my current weight

-500

_____ = Number of calories I should eat each day to lose 1 pound a week

Why a 3500 calorie deficit may not always result in one pound of weight loss.

New research suggests that the human body sometimes adjusts to low-calorie diets. The body is apparently able to do this in two ways: First, it slows down its metabolism.

Secondly, it becomes more efficient at absorbing and storing calories. With repeated dieting, the body becomes really good at adjusting to lower calorie diets, and losing weight becomes harder and harder.

What does this mean for people who are trying to lose weight? It means that if they repeatedly lose and then regain weight, it is going to become more and more difficult for them to lose weight. Thus it is important to lose weight and keep it off permanently rather than go through repeated cycles of dieting and regaining.

You may not even be where you started.

Another rather distressing fact is that when most people regain the weight they have lost by dieting, they usually gain a small additional amount, so they actually end up weighing more than when they began dieting. These small incremental gains in weight can add up over years of cyclical dieting **and** regaining, and leave people worse off **than** if they had never dieted!

This is why it is so important that dieting be taken seriously, with the intent of losing weight permanently once and for all.

How is a calorie like a dime?

You might find it helpful to think of calories as money. Let's say you have a part-time job to earn your spending money. Each week you collect your paycheck. Out of that paycheck you have to pay for lunches, buy your clothes, put gas in the car, get tickets for the movies, and so on. In other words, there are lots of ways to spend that money, and you've got to figure out how to get the most out of it.

It's the same way with calories. You've got a certain number of calories a day to spend. You've got to get your meals and snacks with those calories. And you don't just want the calories, you want to get the nutrients needed for good health along with the calories.

That means you've got to "buy" foods with protein, fat, carbohydrates, vitamins and minerals. Unfortunately a lot of foods have calories from fat and carbohydrate but not much in the way of these other nutrients. You can end up spending all of your calories on these foods without getting nutrients needed for good health.

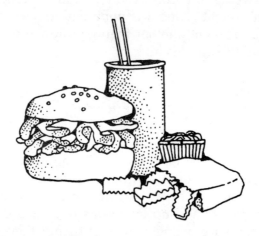

Don't spend all of your calories at one meal.

It's amazing how easily you can manage to use up your calorie allowance without even realizing it:

Quarter pound hamburger with cheese	520 calories
Large serving of french fries	420 calories
Chocolate milk shake	360 calories
Apple pie (single serving dessert size)	300 calories
TOTAL	1600

Have you ever done this? You spent all your calories, and you only had one meal. Most important, you didn't get enough of all the nutrients needed for good health.

% of U.S. RDA's provided by a meal that includes a quarter pound hamburger with cheese, large serving of french fries, a chocolate milk shake, and a single serving of apple pie.

NUTRIENT	% OF U.S. RDA	NUTRIENT	% OF U.S. RDA
Protein	90	Vitamin B-6	45
Vitamin A	20	Folic Acid	6
Vitamin C	64	Vitamin B-12	50
Thiamine	55	Phosphorus	70
Riboflavin	86	Iodine	266
Niacin	126	Magnesium	39
Calcium	60	Zinc	35
Iron	36	Copper	17
Vitamin D	15	Pantothenic Acid	30
Vitamin E	8		

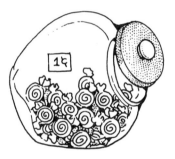

I'd give my right arm for a candy bar.

You've probably seen diets with lists of "NO NO" foods. You aren't supposed to have any candy, potato chips, french fries, cookies, doughnuts, cakes, whip cream, soda, milk shakes, sundaes, and chocolate. The problem is you yearn for these foods. All of a sudden you're dying for a candy bar, or you'd give away your stereo for a bag of potato chips.

It's really OK to have these foods once in awhile; what's not OK is to eat this stuff for breakfast, lunch, dinner, and snacks. Go ahead and eat these foods occasionally; you'll probably be happier with yourself and your attempts at losing weight. But remember, these foods have lots of calories and little in the way of nutrients. If you "spend" too much on them you'll end up overweight and undernourished.

I didn't really have that much.

How much did you really have? How big was the hamburger? How large was the slice of pie? All servings are not equal. One way to control the number of calories you eat is to control the amount of food you put on your plate. Instead of changing the food you eat, change the amount. Do you usually eat a whole baked potato? Next time have just half. Do you like to drink a glass of soda with your pizza? Next time share the soda with a pal. Measure out just one scoop of ice cream instead of casually piling it into the dish.

Can you pick the correct serving size* for foods from each of the Four Food Groups? Try it and see how knowledgeable you are about portions. (See answers at bottom of page 65.)

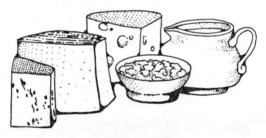

MILK GROUP

Teens need 4 servings a day, adults need 2 servings.

A serving from the milk group is?
½ cup of milk
A 6-ounce glass of milk
An 8-ounce glass of milk

* The standard portions used by governmental agencies.

MEAT GROUP

Teens should try to have 2 servings a day.

A serving from the meat group is?
3 ounces of lean meat, fish, or poultry
6 ounces of lean meat, fish, or poultry
½ pound of lean meat, fish, or poultry

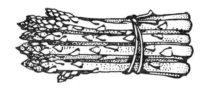

VEGETABLE-FRUIT GROUP

Teens should try to have 4 servings per day.

A serving from the vegetable-fruit group is?
¼ cup vegetable
½ cup vegetable
1 cup vegetable

BREAD-CEREAL GROUP

Teens should try to have 4 servings per day.

A serving from the bread-cereal group is?
½ slice bread
1 slice bread
2 slices bread

[ANSWERS: Milk: An 8 ounce glass. Meat: 3 ounces. Vegetable-Fruit: ½ cup. Bread-Cereal: 1 slice.]

OK, I'm going to try to cut calories;
how do I do it?

Somebody somewhere has probably written a book entitled, "1001 Ways to Cut Calories," but just in case you can't find it, here is your own handy dandy checklist. Look it over. Check the calorie cutting ideas you would like to try. Then use the "calendar" game to plan the days you are going to put the calorie cutting ideas into action. Draw a star in red pen on the days you use one of these ideas. Give yourself two stars if you use two ideas, and so on.

7 important ways to cut calories.
(One for each day of the week)

▶ Bake, broil, or boil instead of frying food. One tablespoon of oil, butter, or margarine adds 100 calories! Look at the differences:

1 plain baked potato	145 calories
10 french fries	214 calories
1 cup hashed brown potatoes	345 calories

▶ Trim the fat off meat before cooking. Fat has more than twice as many calories per gram as protein or carbohydrate.

3 ounces lean pot roast	168 calories
3 ounces pot roast with fat	245 calories

▶ Buy or make your own low-calorie salad dressing.

1 tablespoon diet or low-calorie French dressing	15 calories
1 tablespoon regular French dressing	66 calories

▶ Drink non-fat or low-fat milk instead of whole milk. Use non-fat or low-fat milk when cooking instead of whole milk.

1 glass (8 ounces) non-fat (skim) milk	90 calories
1 glass (8 ounces) 2% low-fat milk	125 calories
1 glass (8 ounces) whole milk	150 calories

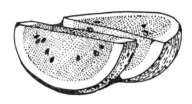

▶ Use fresh fruit for dessert or snacks. Water packed fruit is often sold as dietetic or diet fruit and costs more than fruit packed in syrup, but fruit packed in syrup is loaded with calories.

1 fresh whole peach	40 calories
1 cup canned peach slices in heavy syrup	200 calories
1 slice of peach pie (⅐ of pie)	345 calories

▶ Use herbs and spices for seasoning instead of butter, margarine or sauces.

1 teaspoon spice or herb	1 to 9 calories
1 tablespoon fresh parsley	2 calories
1 tablespoon lemon juice	5 calories
1 tablespoon mustard	12 calories
1 tablespoon sour cream	25 calories
1 tablespoon hollandaise sauce	50 calories
1 tablespoon butter or margarine	100 calories

► Choose low calorie snacks instead of high calorie nibbles.

10 thin pretzel sticks	23 calories
1 cup unbuttered popcorn	25 calories
1 orange	65 calories
1 apple	80 calories
1 chocolate candy bar	145 calories
15 potato chips	170 calories
1 hot fudge sundae	500+ calories

Keep score.

Draw a star with a red pen on each day you use a "calorie cutting" idea.

	Monday	Tuesday	Wednesday	Thursday	Friday	Saturday	Sunday
Week #1							
Week #2							
Week #3							
Week #4							

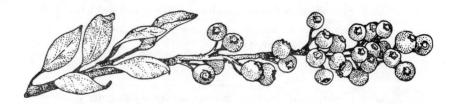

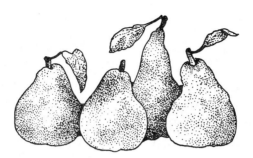

It's time to test my skills.

Now that you know a little about calories and servings, can you cut 500 calories off this teenager's diet for one day? How about 800?

BREAKFAST ON-THE-RUN

peanut butter and jelly sandwich	360 calories
2 tablespoons peanut butter	180 calories
1 tablespoon jelly	50 calories
2 slices whole wheat bread	130 calories
orange	65 calories

LUNCH

cheeseburger	450 calories
3 ounces hamburger meat	235 calories
1 bun	119 calories
1 slice cheddar cheese	96 calories
10 french fries	214 calories
12-ounce cola drink	145 calories

SNACK

10 Cheese-its®	150 calories
1 apple	80 calories

DINNER

1 cup beef vegetable stew	218 calories
salad	151 calories
4 lettuce leaves	12 calories
1 medium tomato	39 calories
1 tablespoon mayonnaise	100 calories
1 slice whole wheat bread	65 calories
1 teaspoon butter	33 calories
1 piece chocolate cake with icing	365 calories
1 8-ounce glass milk	150 calories

SNACK

12 ounces ginger ale	115 calories
1 chocolate brownie	86 calories

One Day's Total Calories	2689

Some ideas — I have lots of my own.

BREAKFAST

Peanut butter has plenty of calories. Why not have a cheese sandwich instead? This eliminates the jelly too, for a total saving of 134 calories.

LUNCH

How about a plain hamburger instead of a cheese-burger? You ate the cheese at breakfast! Substitute a half cup of cole slaw for the french fries. It's lower in calories, 85 as compared to 214, and has more nutrients. How about a glass of skim milk instead of the cola drink? If you make all of those changes, you can eat 530 calories instead of 809, saving a total of 279 calories at lunch.

SNACK

Would just one snack do? Or a lighter snack without the Cheese-its® ?

DINNER

Get a load of the calories in that chocolate cake. Nix that and select from 1 cup of fresh strawberries at 55 calories, a half cantaloupe at 80 calories, or a pear at 100 calories. You can have skim milk instead of whole and save another 60 calories.

SNACK

So far you've had 2 glasses of milk. How about one more in place of the soda? After all, you're a growing teenager and need the calcium that soda won't give you. OK, you can have the brownie if you like, but the 86–calorie brownie measures 1¾ by 1¾ inches and is ⅞ inch thick. Get out your ruler. If it's bigger than that, you're eating more than 86 calories.

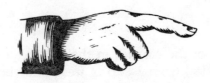

You Are Ready To Go On To Chapter Six
IF:

_____ You have figured out the number of calories you should eat daily in order to lose 1 pound a week.

_____ You have decided which ways you will begin reducing the number of calories you eat.

_____ You figured out how to cut 500 to 800 calories from a day's diet.

_____ **You are continuing with your plans to change your food habits.** (If not, go back to Chapter 2 and start again!)

6

There Must Be
A Quick And Easy Way
To Lose Weight

There must be a secret to losing weight.

"There just has to be an easy way to lose weight! Maybe if I take a pill, get a shot, buy a gadget, try some new diet, I'll lose all I need to lose and keep it off. I'll keep searching, and some day I'll find the secret."

Sound familiar? It should. Everyone is searching for the magic answer. No one has ever counted all the diets that have been published or spread by word-of-mouth, but there must be thousands. Diets make the "best seller" list. They appear in magazines and newspapers. They are a topic of conversation on talk shows and in homes.

Why are people so interested in diets? Because they want to lose weight as quickly and easily as possible. They would all like to lose 20 pounds in two weeks without changing their eating or exercising habits. It's looking for the pot of gold at the end of the rainbow: You know it doesn't exist, but you keep hoping you will be the one to find it.

It isn't hard to find someone ready to offer it: "Try this, buy that, read this, do that, and you'll lose quickly and easily." None of them works. Why? Because there is no quick and easy way to lose weight. Losing weight and keeping it off is hard work — but it helps if you view it as a challenge you are ready to meet.

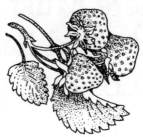

But my friend (enemy, dance instructor, hair stylist, etc.) told me about...

APPETITE CONTROL PILLS

Doctors are reluctant to prescribe appetite suppressants. They realize these pills work for awhile and then lose their effect. Because many of the pills contain amphetamines, a person can become addicted to them.

THE NEW WEIGHT LOSS DISCOVERY

You've seen the full page newspaper ads: "Amazing New Scientific Discovery Allows You to Lose Weight Quickly and Effortlessly — Send in $29.95 for a 30-day supply. Your money back if not satisfied."

Sounds reasonable, doesn't it, especially when they offer to give you your money back. But ask yourself, "Why isn't this amazing new discovery featured on the front page of the newspaper as a

news story instead of in a paid advertisement?"
After all, it would surely be big news if scientists
had discovered an amazing new substance that
melted fat away.

Most of these so-called new scientific discoveries
are substances that scientists have known about for
decades, with no evidence of usefulness in weight
reduction. (Examples include: ornithine and argen-
ine, non-essential amino acids the body synthesizes
on its own; lecithan, a phospholipid that is also not
essential in the diet; cholecystokinin, a hormone the
body produces; and HCG (human corionic gonado-
tropin), a hormone produced in pregnant women.)
Most of these substances are harmful only in that
they create false expectations; none of them causes
weight loss.

So why do these ads appear consistently in major
newspapers? Because by the time the Food and
Drug Administration or U.S. Postal Service takes
action, the promoters have taken their money and
moved on, leaving no forwarding address.

LOW-CARBOHYDRATE DIETS

(Dr. Atkins, Dr. Stillman, "Air Force,"
Quick Weight Loss, Scarsdale)

High-fat, low-carbohydrate diets trigger an abnormal
body response called ketosis, which has been known
to cause fatigue, apathy, dehydration, calcium deple-
tion, kidney trouble, and elevations of blood lipids
associated with heart disease. They can promote a
quick, temporary weight loss, by acting as a diuretic
— but when the water stores are replenished, as
they must be, the weight is back where it started.
Very simply, these are not healthy, well-balanced
diets, and may lead to dangerous side effects.

DIET GROUPS
(Weight Watchers, TOPS, Diet Workshop)

On the whole, people who belong to diet groups are more successful at losing weight than people who try to lose on their own. The group offers each person encouragement, praise, and sympathy. If the idea of joining an already organized group does not appeal to you — you could gather some overweight friends and form a group of your own, each member using a personal copy of this book.

LIQUID FORMULA DIETS
(Metrecal, Slender)

Liquid formula diets come in cans and are usually sold in supermarkets. Although nutritious, they lack fiber and if they are the sole food, constipation may become a problem. Many people find drinking all of their meals for weeks monotonous and boring. Only use them occasionally as a meal substitute.

THE SPECIAL FOOD, FOOD GROUP, OR FOOD COMBINATIONS
(Fit for Life, Beverly Hills, Mayo Clinic, Grapefruit, Grapefruit and Egg)

There is no food, food group, or food combination that will help your body "burn fat," "move fat cells out of the body," or "fully digest food so you won't get fat." (Actually, just the opposite is true; fully digested food contributes calories that can end up as body fat.) The creators of these diets also create their own rules of biochemistry — rules that don't work scientifically. If you have questions about strange-sounding claims, talk to your science teacher about them. He or she will probably tell you, "No, that is not how the human body actually functions."

EXERCISE GADGETS, BODY WRAPS, POTIONS, CELLULITE REMOVERS

(Bicycles, flexible lounge chairs, slant boards, lotions, vibrators, sweatsuits, figure wrapping)

These products are often promoted as "passive weight reduction" methods. This means that you don't do a thing except to sit or lie on it or in it, wear it, or rub it in. But, you can't massage, jiggle, sweat, beat, stroke, or melt fat away. The only items on this list that have the potential of helping you lose weight are the exercise gadgets, and they are useful only if you are the one who is exercising and not the gadget!

FASTING

(starvation)

Fasting can be a dangerous way to lose weight. Total fasting (with carefully monitored vitamin/mineral supplementation) is occasionally used as a "last resort" for dangerously obese patients — under close medical supervision. No person, no matter how overweight and desperate, should attempt total fasting on his/her own.

MODIFIED FAST

(Cambridge, Optifast, other)

Under the close supervision of a competent physician, the modified fast is an acceptable way of losing weight. Without close medical supervision, however, it can have serious effects on health, such as altering body chemistry, weakness and fainting, and the breakdown of some body tissues. These changes can trigger an assortment of ailments and disorders. See a doctor before (and, of course, during) attempts to use this diet.

Is this diet for me?

Browse in the local bookstore, leaf through the latest issue of a fashion magazine, check the newspaper. Everywhere you look there are diets. Your friends ask you to go to a diet group with them. Your relatives are eager to tell you about the "Ice Cream Lover's Diet," the "Calorie Counter's Diet," and the "Eat All You Want and Lose Diet." Which ones might really help you lose weight and keep it off?

Here is a checklist guide to evaluating diets. You can use it to judge the worth of any diet you read about, see advertised, or hear of from well-meaning friends and relatives. If any of the statements doesn't hold true for a "diet" you are considering, it probably won't work for you.

Judging diets.

▶ I can stay on this diet for 3 to 6 months.

   Does the diet include foods you like? If it does, it will be much easier for you to stay on it for 3 to 6 months. If you are restricted to eating just a few foods, the diet may become monotonous and boring and you'll be very tempted to forget the whole thing.

▶ I can afford to buy the foods recommended.

   Does the diet suggest you eat steak 3 times a day? Your parents may balk at the idea of spending that much money on food. Some diets suggest you purchase expensive diet foods, pills, or formulas. Are you sure you can afford these items?

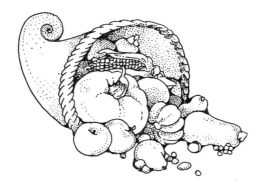

▶ The diet is nutritionally balanced and won't endanger my health.

Does the diet suggest you eat foods from all of The Four Food Groups:

Milk Group: Milk, cheese, cottage cheese, yogurt, pudding, cream soups

Meat Group: Meat, poultry, fish, nuts, eggs, dried peas and beans

Bread-Cereal Group: Bread, cereal, rice, tortillas, flour, cornmeal, pasta

Fruit-Vegetable Group: All fruits and vegetables

By eating a variety of foods from each of The Four Food Groups, you will get the nutrients you need for good health.

▶ I will be eating at least 3 times a day and possibly up to 5 times.

Research has shown that successful dieters tend to eat 3 to 5 times a day, while unsuccessful dieters eat 2 or fewer times a day. Eating more frequently will help you avoid binges.

▶ I will be eating fewer calories than I usually do and/or I will be getting more exercise.

Unless the above statement is true, there is no way you can start to lose weight.

▶ I will learn some low-calorie ways of preparing and selecting food.

Does the diet give you some practical advice on how to cut calories? If it does, you may find the tips and hints useful for the rest of your life.

▶ I will lose one to two pounds a week on this diet.

The best way to lose weight is slowly. You may not always lose steadily. One week you may lose three pounds and then not lose any weight for two weeks, then lose again. Rapid weight loss can endanger your health. Often it is just a result of body water loss, that is regained later.

▶ I will permanently change my food and exercise habits as a result of this diet.

When people go on "diets," they expect that after they have lost weight they will be able to go off the diet and eat normally again. This usually results in their gaining back all the weight they lost. In order to lose weight and keep it off, it is necessary to permanently change one's eating and exercising habits. See Chapter 2 for advice on how to do this.

Let me be the judge of this.

Here are three diets. Using the "Judging diets" checklist, see if you can think of reasons why each diet would or would not help a person to lose weight and keep it off.

THE ROCK STAR'S SECRET DIET

How does the incredibly popular rock star stay incredibly thin? It's easy, just by eating from two food groups. Choose any foods from the Fruit-Vegetable Food Group or from the Bread and Cereal Food Group, but be sure to emphasize choices high in fiber and complex carbohydrates. These foods will help clean out your digestive tract. Whatever you do, don't eat foods from the Milk and Milk Product Food Group or the Meat, Fish, Poultry, Eggs Food Group. These are loaded with poisons like fat and cholesterol, and will up your weight for sure.

THE BICYCLE LOVER'S DIET

You can continue to eat most of the foods you have been eating with some limitations. You cannot consume more that a half cup of each of any three foods at a meal. You are allowed to eat three meals a day and one fresh fruit snack. You must spend at least a half hour every day riding your bike. (This diet was in the *Biker's Digest* magazine.)

THE "MAGIC CANDY" DIET

You can eat as much as you want of anything you want any time you want. Before eating any food you must eat a piece of the "magic candy" you purchase at the local drugstore. If the candy is not available, eat a lifesaver instead. (This diet has been advertised on television.)

The expert's comments — compare them to yours.

THE ROCK STAR'S SECRET DIET

Watch the rock star suffer from malnutrition! His diet is low in calcium, protein, and a host of other nutrients. The advice about eating foods high in fiber and complex carbohydrates is fine. Foods high in fiber do aid in digestion. However, there are many low-fat, low-cholesterol food choices in the Milk and Milk Products Food Group as well as in the Meat, Fish, Poultry, Eggs Food Group, and these food groups provide essential nutrients necessary for health and growth.

THE BICYCLE LOVER'S DIET

Allows a variety of food. Limits portion sizes. May permanently change exercise habits. Could work!

THE "MAGIC CANDY" DIET

A waste of money. Doesn't encourage a person to eat fewer calories or exercise more in order to lose weight. Won't lead to changed eating or exercise habits.

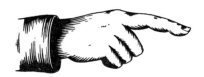

You Are Ready To Go On To Chapter Seven
IF:

_____ You can judge the worth of diets you read or hear about.

_____ **You are continuing with your plans to change your food habits.**

7

Temptation Is Knocking At My Lips

It's party time.

There's nothing like a party to ruin good intentions. You're doing so well, and then along come bowls of potato chips, bags of pretzels, plates of pizza, and all sorts of tempting goodies. What's a person to do?

First use your imagination. Literally. Before the party sit down and daydream that you are already at the party. *Who else is there? What record is playing? Now, imagine you see the food. There's a whole table covered with your favorite snacks. Walk over to it and take a good look. Really check it out. Decide exactly what you are going to eat during the evening. Say to yourself, "I'll eat 10 potato chips, but no dip. I'll have about a cup of popcorn. Since there's no diet soda, I better remember to bring a can." Now you're walking away from the table. You're standing on the other side of the room. You know that you better not stand next to the food — after all, you're only human. Suddenly a pushy person comes up and shoves a dish of nuts in your hand. You say, "No thanks. I'll help myself if I want something." You offer to serve the pizza so you can give yourself a small portion without having to refuse a large serving offered to you. On the way home, you compliment yourself on how well you did!* End of daydream.

What you are doing is mentally rehearsing your behavior at the party. When you really go to the party, you'll have already been there in your imagination. You'll know how you're going to handle things. You'll be in control. And on the way home, you will be able to congratulate yourself!

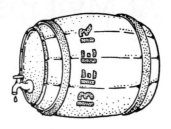

Can I drink and still lose weight?

Some people think alcohol doesn't have any calories so it can't make you fat. But that isn't so! Alcohol has 7 calories to the gram. (Protein and carbohydrate have 4 calories to the gram and fat has 9 calories per gram.) What does all this calorie and gram business mean in terms of real drinks? Here is the low down:

DRINK	NUMBER OF CALORIES
Ale (12 oz.)	225
Beer (12 oz.)	165
Gin (1½ oz.)	126
Whiskey (1½ oz.)	112
Vodka (1½ oz.)	135
Daiquiri (2¼ oz. rum)	180
Manhattan (2¼ oz. whiskey)	200

DRINK	NUMBER OF CALORIES
Martini (2¼ oz. gin)	220
Dry champagne (1 champagne glass, approx. 5 oz.)	105
Sweet champagne (1 glass, 5 oz.)	160
Red wine (claret glass, 4 oz.)	100
White wine (4 oz.)	95
Port, sherry (sherry glass, 2 oz.)	100

Just in case those calories don't impress you very much, try thinking of it this way: If you drink just one 12-ounce beer every day for a month, you'll be taking in enough calories to put on about 2 pounds. Needless to say, if you want to lose weight, you have to limit drinking.

The grass that isn't green.

Marijuana is a known appetite stimulant. When you're high, food flavors are accentuated. All your favorite foods taste terrific. When you've got the munchies, you want to eat, eat, eat. And you do, do, do. Be aware.

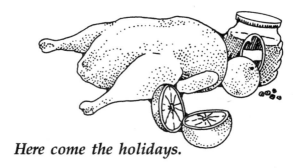

Here come the holidays.

Trick or treat candy at Halloween...turkey and trimmings on Thanksgiving...cookies and candy canes at Christmas...boxes of chocolates on Valentine's day. It's never ending. How will you cope? One idea is to start keeping your food diary again. You may find that you've reverted back to your old food habits. The food diary will help you see where you've gotten out of line.

Start setting some specific goals for yourself and decide how you're going to achieve them. You may find that food is all too available during holidays. Can you get some of it behind cupboard doors? Can you avoid going into the kitchen? You may be eating irregularly again. Start keeping a calendar to get yourself back on the three-meal-a-day pattern. Remember, when your Easter bunny costume feels a little too snug, or your Santa suit doesn't fit any more, it's time to go back to Chapter 2 and refresh your memory.

It's just baby fat, my dear.

There she is, your dear sweet grandmother (godmother, aunt, mother) who loves you just the way you are. And the way you are is fat. She doesn't think you need to lose weight. She makes your favorite dessert and urges you to eat, eat, eat. She grew up in an age when "fat" equalled "healthy." Now we know better. But it's difficult to get the message across to her. Nonetheless you've got to try. The first thing to do is to tell her how she can help you.

Dear Grandma,

Please don't offer me food. I'll ask for something when I get hungry.

Please don't urge me to have seconds or eat more than what I've served myself. I need to take control of my eating.

I would really like a shirt (one size smaller than I wear now) for my birthday instead of a box of candy or dinner at a fancy restaurant.

Can we keep food behind cupboard doors? If it's sitting out on counters or around the house, I may not be able to resist eating it.

Please let me initiate any conversations about losing weight. This is a sensitive subject with me.

Can you praise me for my efforts to lose weight, and ignore me when I'm not doing what I should?

I'd prefer it if we don't tell anyone about my plans to lose weight. I'd like to surprise people in a few months.

Thanking you with love,

You may find the same approach works well with overanxious parents. They may be coming from the opposite direction — they're too eager for you to lose weight and are constantly nagging you about it. Let them know that you are trying to change your weight, and you'll need help from them. Give them the same list of requests!

Eating out is a special trip.

Eating in restaurants presents new temptations. You find yourself feeling guilty if you don't eat everything — and you find yourself feeling just as guilty when you do! Your conscience says, "Clean your plate. People in North Africa are starving!" Then it says, "You're on a diet. You should resist overeating." The people you're with may add their two cents, and ask if you're going to leave all that food after paying "good" money for it. You don't know what to do.

Take the advice of the skinny gourmet:

The secrets of checking out the menu and ordering.

- ► Look for main dishes that are baked or boiled.
- ► Skip anything that is served with sauce or gravy.
- ► If french fries are served with the item you want, ask if you can substitute a baked potato or rice.

► Order the salad dressing on the side so you can decide how much to put on. Forget the bleu cheese or roquefort, ask for low-calorie or oil and vinegar. Go easy on the oil and heavy on the vinegar.

► Ask if the fruit salad is made with fresh fruit. If so, you might want to try it. If it's made with canned fruit packed in heavy syrup, it's overloaded with extra calories.

► Be skeptical of "diet plates." Some are actually higher in calories than other menu items. A half pound of ground beef, half cup of cottage cheese, and sliced tomato add up to almost 800 calories.

► If the dish has a fancy name and you're not sure exactly what it is or how it's made, flatter the waiter or waitress by asking them about it.

► Specifically ask for small portions when you order.

The secret of not overeating when the food has arrived.

► Ask the waiter or waitress for an empty plate. Portion off food you don't want to be tempted to eat onto the plate and ask that it be removed. Or, portion off the amount of food you don't want to eat and put enough sugar or salt on it so it's inedible and you won't be tempted to eat it.

► Let the rolls and butter sit at the other end of the table.

► Politely refuse the menu when the waiter or waitress offers it for desserts. Ask if they have fresh fruit. Order something like a dish of strawberries if you want dessert.

► Remind yourself that you're not just paying for the food at the restaurant. You're paying for the service of having somebody else cook the food, serve it, and clean up afterwards. Even if you don't eat everything, you're still getting your money's worth.

► Ask for a "doggie bag" even if you don't have a doggie. You can take the leftovers for another day.

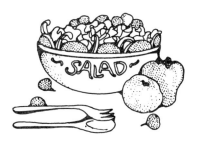

What does the skinny gourmet advise about fast foods?

► Order a taco or plain hamburger.

► Skip fried foods like french fries, fried chicken, and potato chips.

► Cole slaw is a good choice as a side dish.

► Milkshakes are high in calories. Soda is lower but a poor choice in terms of nutrition. Your best bet is a carton of milk. If it's low-fat or skim milk, that's to your advantage. If you've got to have the shake, halve the calories by sharing it with a friend.

► Bring a banana, orange, apple, or other fresh fruit from home for dessert.

► Try the salad bar but go easy on the dressing.

They do it all for you.

Eating out doesn't always mean fancy restaurants. More often than not, it's McDonald's or Burger King. The biggest problem with fast food is that it tends to be loaded with calories. You'll have to be selective if you're trying to stay within a calorie limit.

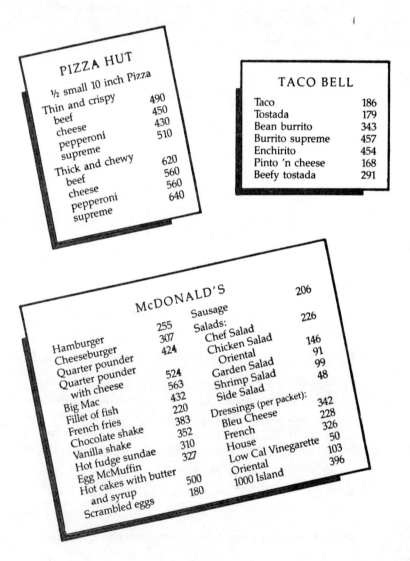

PIZZA HUT

½ small 10 inch Pizza

Thin and crispy

beef	490
cheese	450
pepperoni	430
supreme	510

Thick and chewy

beef	620
cheese	560
pepperoni	560
supreme	640

TACO BELL

Taco	186
Tostada	179
Bean burrito	343
Burrito supreme	457
Enchirito	454
Pinto 'n cheese	168
Beefy tostada	291

McDONALD'S

Hamburger	255	Sausage	206
Cheeseburger	307	Salads:	
Quarter pounder	424	Chef Salad	226
Quarter pounder		Chicken Salad	146
with cheese	524	Oriental	91
Big Mac	563	Garden Salad	99
Fillet of fish	432	Shrimp Salad	48
French fries	220	Side Salad	
Chocolate shake	383	Dressings (per packet):	
Vanilla shake	352	Bleu Cheese	342
Hot fudge sundae	310	French	228
Egg McMuffin	327	House	326
Hot cakes with butter		Low Cal Vinegarette	50
and syrup	500	Oriental	103
Scrambled eggs	180	1000 Island	396

DAIRY QUEEN

Small cone	110
Small malt	340
Small sundae	170
Mr. Misty freeze	500

KENTUCKY FRIED CHICKEN

2-piece dinner, drum and thigh
(includes 2 pieces of chicken, mashed potato and gravy, cole slaw and roll)

original recipe	643
extra crispy	855

WENDY'S

Single hamburger	470
Double hamburger	670
Triple hamburger	850
Single with cheese	580
Double with cheese	800
Triple with cheese	1040
Taco salad	460
Chili	230
French fries	330
Frosty	390

(lettuce, tomato, onion, pickle, mustard and catsup included on all burgers.)

BURGER KING

Whopper	630
Whopper Jr.	370
Double Beef Whopper	850
Whopper with cheese	740
Whopper Jr. with cheese	
Cheeseburger	420
Fries	305
Onion Rings	210
Vanilla shake	270
Chocolate shake	340
Coke (12 oz.)	340
	144

Prepackaged Salads:

Chef Salad	180
Garden Salad	110
Pasta Salad	250
Shrimp Salad	90
Side Salad	20

Dressings (per serving):

Bleu Cheese	
French	300
House	280
Reduced Low-Cal	260
Italian	30
1000 Island	240

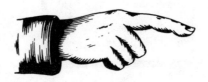

You Are Ready To Go On To Chapter Eight IF:

_____ You have mentally rehearsed how you are going to handle food at a party.

_____ You understand the temptations alcohol and marijuana present to the over-weight person, and you have decided whether, and if so how, to use them.

_____ You know what to do when your eating gets out of hand during the holidays.

_____ You have given your parents and anyone else who influences your eating a list of ways they can be helpful to you as you change your eating habits.

_____ You have practiced ordering from a restaurant or fast food menu.

_____ **You are continuing with your plans to change your food habits.**

8

Rewards For
Good Behavior

Your first step in changing your food habits was to keep the food diary. The food diary has helped you to discover the habits you need to change. The next step has been to plan changes in your behavior. You have set some specific behavioral goals to work towards.

Now there is one more necessary step to include. It is called reinforcement or reward. Your new behaviors will be repeated and strengthened if they are reinforced with a reward. For example, say you practice eating more slowly at lunch. If your parents notice this and compliment you, you are more likely to eat slowly at dinner.

A reward is anything that you enjoy. It may be a compliment from an important other person. It may be an activity or hobby you like. Or, it may be something material like a new record.

It's not a good idea to reward yourself with food when you have a weight problem. That's kind of like rewarding yourself with a cigarette because you've quit smoking. It doesn't work.

You need to reward yourself every time you do something to change your habits. Let's say you start eating lunch because you're trying to get on a three-meal-a-day plan; then reward yourself when you've finished lunch. Or, if you are trying to keep food out of your bedroom, reward yourself after you have removed the food from your room or when you resist taking it there.

It is best to plan your rewards. Then you will feel motivated to carry through on your plans for change, because you'll know something good is going to happen when you do.

Here are some lists of potential rewards. Can you add some of your own personal ideas of rewards to these lists?

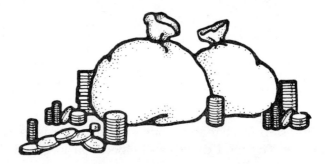

Things I can use to reward myself.

Check the ones that apply to you. Add your own personal rewards to the lists.

Things I like to do that don't cost anything.

_____ Read comic books

_____ Play catch with the dog

_____ Listen to record/ tape/disc

_____ Window shop

_____ Take a bubble bath

_____ Watch a sports event on TV

_____ Play checkers (chess, cards, jacks, scrabble, etc.)

_____ Wear special perfume/aftershave

_____ Solve puzzles

_____ Read mysteries/
science fiction/
romance

_____ Work on the car

_____ Watch my favorite
TV show

_____ Talk on the
telephone

_____ Write to friends

_____ Work on collection
of _____

_____ Manicure
fingernails

_____ Play an instrument

_____ Attend a club
meeting

_____

_____

_____

_____

Things I like to do that may cost something.

_____ Go to the movies

_____ Shoot pool

_____ Visit a museum

_____ See a sports event

_____ Buy a new record/
tape/disc

_____ Get some new
clothes

_____ Sew

_____ Take lessons to
learn to _____

_____ Go out to lunch
with a friend

_____ Have a picnic

_____ Get new sports
equipment

_____ Take an overnight
hike

_____ Have hair done

_____ Golf, ski, swim,
play tennis

_____ Roller skate or ice
skate

_____ Hunt or fish

_____

_____

_____

_____

_____

_____

Thinking the good thoughts.

There may be some situations where you're really hard up for a reward. You just can't use any of the things on the checklist. But there is still a reward that is always available to you at any time. It's a daydream. Sound crazy? It's really not when you think about it. Daydreams are fun. All kinds of marvelously good things can happen to you in your imagination. Why not try it?

First, you need to relax. Let all the tension flow out of your body. Let your mind wander for a few minutes. Don't think about anything in particular. Then start to focus in on a specific daydream you enjoy. You might imagine that you are in the most beautiful place in the world. Wander through it slowly. Enjoy the wonders of it. Your daydream can include romance, adventure, suspense, whatever turns you on. You can think of other daydreams that give you pleasure and use these to reward yourself.

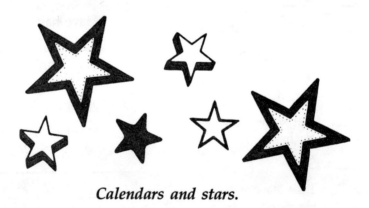

Calendars and stars.

In Chapter 3, it is suggested that you draw red stars on calendars to keep track of your progress in changing your behavior. You might want to use the stars as part of your reward system. For example, 5 stars could be 15 minutes to do something special. 10 stars might mean a reward that costs something. You can post your calendar for others to see so they can compliment you as you fill your calendar with stars.

Money, money, money, money, money, money.

Money is the only reward that is meaningful to some people. It is possible to use money as a self-reward, but you have to have a system to make it work. First, you need to decide how much money you will reward yourself for specific behaviors. You might want to make a list like this:

eating breakfast	$.50 per meal
eating lunch	$.50 per meal
eating only in the kitchen when I'm home	$1.00 per day
eating more slowly at a meal	$.25 per meal
doing something other than eating when I'm hungry	$.50 per hunger period

Then follow through, by rewarding yourslf and setting the specified amount of money aside for something you want. If you neglect to use the money as you had plannned, you must put the same amount in an envelope, address it to your worst enemy or a cause you don't support, and mail it. The threat of losing the money will provide potent motivation to stick to your plans to change your behavior.

The only other system that works is to give the money to someone else who then uses it to reward you for good behavior. If you don't do as you're supposed to, then the person gets to keep the money. You might try this with a brother, sister, friend, or parent. It all depends on how much you want to involve them in your plans for change.

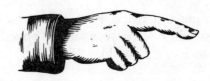

You Are Ready To Go On To Chapter Nine
IF:

_____ You have selected some rewards for yourself.

_____ You are using the rewards to reward yourself for specific behavioral changes in eating and exercising habits.

_____ **You are continuing with your plans to change your food habits.**

9

Keeping It Off

I did it!

You have now changed your shape by changing your eating and exercising habits. By adopting new habits, you've licked your weight problem. That's really exciting. You should feel proud of yourself! Just think of all the good things that have happened to you:

▶ You're eating more regular meals and snacks. As a result, you feel more energetic and alert, especially in mid-morning. You're less tempted to binge, since you don't get as hungry as you used to when you ate irregularly.

▶ You're taking more time to eat your food, and you're enjoying it more. You're experiencing the good taste of everything you eat.

▶ You're not tempted to overeat by the things that happen around you. You've taken control of your eating.

▶ You're moving around more, and you feel a lot better as a result. You're physically fit!

► You know what to do when hunger strikes. Now you can fight back.

► You've found new ways to reward yourself for controlling your eating and exercising.

Contratulations! Those are some big changes to make and they probably took you awhile to accomplish.

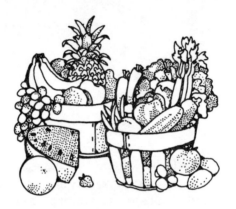

Can I keep it off?

Now that you've achieved your weight loss goal, you're probably wondering if you can keep it off? Sure you can! You've found out which of your habits caused you to be overweight, and you've changed those habits. The new eating and exercising habits you've adopted will help you maintain your weight loss.

What if I start to gain again?

If you find your weight creeping up, start keeping the food diary again. Look it over carefully to discover which of your old food habits has reappeared on the scene. Then it's time to work on those habits, using the same approach suggested in Chapter 3. You did it once and it worked, so try it again. You'll find it just as helpful the second time around.

A pledge to myself.

I have learned new ways of eating and exercising. I must continue to use them, or I will regain the weight I have lost.

I realize there is no "magic" way to lose weight, and that it is a matter of eating less or being more physically active.

Because I have worked so hard at losing weight and have been successful, I won't let myself down by going back to my old habits.

_____

(SIGNATURE)

_____

(DATE)

_____

(CURRENT WEIGHT)

FOOD DIARY

Day _____

Time of Day	Minutes Spent Eating	Places You Eat	Other Activity While Eating	How Hungry You Feel	Mood	Food	Amount	Calories

FOOD DIARY

Day _____

Time of Day	Minutes Spent Eating	Places You Eat	Other Activity While Eating	How Hungry You Feel	Mood	Food	Amount	Calories

FOOD DIARY

Day _____

Time of Day	Minutes Spent Eating	Places You Eat	Other Activity While Eating	How Hungry You Feel	Mood	Food	Amount	Calories

FOOD DIARY

Day ___

Time of Day	Minutes Spent Eating	Places You Eat	Other Activity While Eating	How Hungry You Feel	Mood	Food	Amount	Calories

FOOD DIARY

Day _____

Time of Day	Minutes Spent Eating	Places You Eat	Other Activity While Eating	How Hungry You Feel	Mood	Food	Amount	Calories

FOOD DIARY

Day _____

Time of Day	Minutes Spent Eating	Places You Eat	Other Activity While Eating	How Hungry You Feel	Mood	Food	Amount	Calories

FOOD DIARY   Day ____

Time of Day	Minutes Spent Eating	Places You Eat	Other Activity While Eating	How Hungry You Feel	Mood	Food	Amount	Calories

FOOD DIARY

Day _____

Time of Day	Minutes Spent Eating	Places You Eat	Other Activity While Eating	How Hungry You Feel	Mood	Food	Amount	Calories

FOOD DIARY

Day _____

Time of Day	Minutes Spent Eating	Places You Eat	Other Activity While Eating	How Hungry You Feel	Mood	Food	Amount	Calories